There Is No College in COVID

There Is No College in COVID

in COVID

Selections from the
Oregon State University–Cascades
COVID-19 Journaling Project

First Parafine Press Edition 2021
ISBN: 978-1-950843-52-7

Parafine Press
5322 Fleet Avenue
Cleveland, Ohio 44105
www.parafinepress.com
Cover and book design by Meredith Pangrace

ACKNOWLEDGMENTS

This project was generously supported by a grant from the Oregon State University Women's Giving Circle. All proceeds from the sale of this publication will go toward Oregon State University–Cascades scholarships.

Thanks to Spencer Veatch (U-Engage, Fall '20) who helped with early editorial work and whose entry on October 4, 2020, provided the inspiration for such an evocative title for this book.

Thanks to Interim OSU–Cascades Vice President Andrew Ketsdever for writing a timely and thoughtful foreword for this volume.

Finally, thanks to Teresa Ashford, a partner-in-pandemic.

FOREWORD

"In the end, during our brief moment in the sun, we are tasked with the noble charge of finding our own meaning."

> —Brian Greene, *Until the End of Time: Mind, Matter, and Our Search for Meaning in an Evolving Universe.*

I was appointed Dean of Academic Affairs in July of 2020. It seemed as though I had chosen a completely inappropriate time to take a step up in academic leadership. The COVID-19 global pandemic was (and in a sense still is) in full swing. In March of 2020, we knew, like many other universities, that we would be going remote for winter term final exams and that most courses for the spring term would be delivered in a fully remote modality. Due to directives from the state, we were forced to go fully remote for nearly all of our classes in the spring term of 2020 in the matter of two weeks. We simply were in a mode to survive the upcoming ten-week term.

However, the fall 2020 term was supposed to be different. In effect, we had three months to prepare our fall courses for a remote modality. Presumably, we learned everything we needed to know in the direness of spring term, and fall was looking promising. As fall term approached, the COVID-19 situation did not improve. In many areas, and particularly in Central Oregon, the situation got worse. Our first-year students that missed the last term of high school were now faced with missing in-person experiences in their first term of college. The class ALS 199 was designed as a support course for students in their first term of college to find connection, improve needed skills, and find meaning in their education. The students in ALS 199 simply found themselves in the same boat as nearly everyone else, stuck with the reality that their first college experience was going to be viewed through a two-dimensional screen attached to an electronic device.

This book is a collection of journal entries from first-year, first-term students in ALS 199 from the fall term in 2020. These journal entries lead to deep reflection about the experiences of these first-term college students. The sum weight of the entries in this book is impressive, overwhelming, and downright sad all at once. How will we reconcile these experiences and our decisions should we be put in this unfortunate situation again? That is where this book has its roots and where it finds its meaning.

I didn't expect that this book would reflect many of the decisions that I had to make as a new dean from the perspective of these students, yet there they are. As I look back today, I feel that we provided students with an "all things considered" amazing experience during the pandemic. Our small class sizes and more intimate interactions with faculty and peers certainly helped during the pandemic, but there are other factors such as encouraging more community that we could have emphasized more.

Due to the keen foresight of Dr. Jenna Goldsmith, this collection was saved as a memorial to the first-year student experience in the face of a global pandemic. Elliana B. commented near the end of the term that she "started college during a global pandemic. How many people can say that?" Dr. Goldsmith is an amazing writer in her own right, and she certainly brings out the best in her students, as you will see throughout their entries.

The students' thoughts show a similar progression throughout the term that many of us felt, yet their perspectives during this unique time in their lives is highly insightful. We begin to understand the thoughts of living away from home for the first time in this situation. We see the impacts of being asked to test for COVID-19, to quarantine, and to study. We gain some insight into the decisions to go home for holidays to see loved ones or to shelter in place instead.

At the start of the fall term, Spencer V. commented, "College is not just academia; it is a community." Somehow the fully remote scenario that he found himself in did not translate. It was delivering on the academics but lacked the sense of community that was critical too. Lucy F. wrote, "It's almost like the school year is just happening to me." There was a general feeling of a lack of control over the situation—that action was futile, and the approach was to sit back and watch as things unfolded.

When you read "COVID-19 Poem" by Gulian C. and the journal entry of Susan G., your heart will simply break. The global pandemic hit students hard and close to home.

We see fear as the pandemic pressed on without an end in sight. William W. wrote, "I worry that our campus will close," and Frances R. reveals, "As we enter a statewide freeze, I am starting to become stressed and unsure of what life might look like in a month or so." As the term wraps up, we see some self-realization and the willingness to provide ourselves some grace. Gulian C. wrote, "Good job Gulian," a clear indication that she survived and did her best. As the term wrapped up, Alexandria M. put it best: "I just want normal back."

I am grateful and honored to be asked to write this foreword. My thoughts echo in the comments of Frances R., "When looking back (on my experiences), I notice a lot of growth and self-realization."

Andrew D. Ketsdever, Ph.D.
Interim Vice President
Oregon State University–Cascades
August 2021

INTRODUCTION

For some time, Oregon State University–Cascades, a small branch campus located in Bend, has offered a course called ALS 199, affectionately named "U-Engage." U-Engage is an elective course for first-term, first-year students who want a bit of extra support at the start of their college journey. Through class visitors and guest lecturers, students enjoy a direct line to chairs of programs and departments on campus, career development specialists, advisors, diversity and equity coordinators, school counselors, and health advisors, in addition to other campus staff and faculty who could make their time with us more informed, more safe, and of course, more fun. I became the resident U-Engage instructor when I arrived on campus in the fall of 2016, relishing the opportunity to welcome new students to campus. I appreciated the latitude the university afforded me in crafting a meaningful experience for students that, I felt, got them off on the right foot. I often told others that, had U-Engage been offered at the college I attended in my first year, I would have enrolled.

Despite the practicality and adaptability of the course, our main campus counterparts decided to discontinue the U-Engage program. On our campus, advisors and administrators witnessed how effective U-Engage was to student learning and retention, so we went rogue and kept a section. I was relieved. Even before the pandemic pushed us into more isolated environments—and despite the seemingly endless array of social apps available to them—students seemed to be experiencing college in increasingly cloistered ways. Witnessing this firsthand, I decided to make *connection* the cornerstone of my U-Engage courses. I wanted students to have a chance to meet (and maybe even get to know) folks on campus they would otherwise not have cause to engage.

In a spin on the *Humans of New York* project spearheaded by photojournalist Brandon Stanton in 2010, wherein Stanton gathered photos and quotes from everyday New Yorkers and posted them to the world through his blog, I developed a similar project called *Humans of OSU–Cascades* for Instagram (@humansofosucascades). Every week, pairs of students found interviewees (this could be anyone associated with OSU–Cascades), secured permission to use their photo and words, and conducted interviews. I edited the interview snippets for clarity and posted the pieces to the Instagram account each week. Between the fall of 2016 and the fall of 2019, we posted 274 times. Each post signaled an interaction, a possible connection the students might not have had otherwise. I was tickled to learn of a few love connections forged during these interviews. Mission accomplished.

I felt that I had hit the pedagogical jackpot with this assignment. Students loved it because it challenged them to branch out. Administrators loved it because it gained some notoriety and was free content for the official university social media platforms. And personally, I enjoyed facilitating the whole experience. In the process, it helped me learn a fair amount about the students, staff, and faculty on my new campus.

From there, the story took a now foreseeable detour. Forced to move U-Engage online in the fall of 2020 because of the COVID-19 pandemic, I needed to pivot. (I promised myself and others I would never again use this word outside of a basketball court, and yet here I am.) How could I teach a class centered on connection without the connection piece? How could I capture the spirit of U-Engage and the *Humans of OSU–Cascades* project in a remote setting like Zoomland?

Though finding creative ways to connect with one another would become crucial to our well-being during the pandemic, I also felt that reconnecting with ourselves— avoiding the mindlessness of doom-scrolling, tapping into the basics of self-care, returning to or learning new solitary hobbies and interests—was key. So, instead of having students interview others, I assigned students a project that required them to interview themselves . . . sort of. I called it the COVID-19 Journaling Project. The assignment was simple: write two journal entries twice a week of any length about your experience as a college student during a global pandemic. If an entry felt too personal for a possible wider audience down the road (this publication, for instance), students could mark the entry as such and it would only exist in the space of our class. The entries willingly put forth by students are deeply personal explorations of the meaning of college during a pandemic.

So that some of the details of these entries may be understood in context, it feels important to provide readers with a bit of explanation. First, as you read, you will notice some students were living in our university's residence hall, while others sheltered in place. Those who remained at home did so to take care of children and/or elders, to minimize housing costs, or to keep their potential exposure to a minimum. Additionally, some will remember the horrendous wildfires that blanketed the west coast in the fall of 2020; the smoke from these fires appear in these entries as well. Just when we needed it most, the dangerous air quality removed the outdoors as an option for recreation and gathering. Finally, the entries appear chronologically and have been edited for clarity but are otherwise original in tone and sentiment.

In this selection of entries, there exists a wide array of position, analysis, and opinion regarding the students' observations. This serves to create a compelling cross-section of our community's response to the COVID-19 pandemic. We witness frustration in these accounts, sadness over the loss of family and friends, appreciation for the simple pleasures in life, and confusion about what would come next. Collectively, what the students have in common is their station as first-term, first-year students grappling with the uncertainty and significant disruption brought about by an unprecedented global pandemic.

I have since left OSU–Cascades for another university and will likely never meet these students in person; our interactions were limited to Zoom and phone calls. It was my honor to engage with them for a term, to read their stories, and to publish their voices here. This volume is for all college students who started college in the COVID-19 global pandemic.

Jenna Goldsmith, PhD
Bloomington, Illinois
July 2021

There Is No College in COVID

When I was a kid and would think about college, I had always imagined a setting where there were lots of social activities and nonstop fun. COVID has put a massive brace on this metaphor of college; the idea of masks and social distancing just didn't sound like a college experience for me. This has made me even more happy to have chosen Bend as my college destination. If I had gone to Corvallis, I would be thinking about big groups of people and living the full college experience, which obviously isn't possible these days. The pandemic had put a big setback in all of our social lives, after not talking to anyone for so long it was difficult to get back in the rhythm. For a good three months, we all spent our lives sheltered, only talking to friends on video games or FaceTime. This made me and other people I know truly find out who cares for them in their lives. To wrap up my thoughts on the whole COVID experience, it has been the weirdest, scariest and craziest time in my life.

Colin B.
September 28, 2020

Today I truly felt the trapped, stuck feeling a lot of people have been describing due to COVID, especially students. I had two Zoom classes today, each lasting about 1½ to 2 hours long. Sitting in my desk chair for that long Monday through Thursday is making me realize how much of my normal life I'm missing out on: seeing friends in classes and talking to them, going out for lunch at the nearest fast-food restaurant; walking through the halls and having those small head nods and smiles and waves at people I know; engaging with each teacher and classroom in-person has a certain charisma that sadly Zoom can't completely fulfill. Today I sat for hours without even getting up, or hardly moving, really. I felt so bored and so upset and claustrophobic. But I know that we are all in this together and there's not much I can do about it.

Maybe I'll try a different setting next time and see how that goes.

Hanna S.
September 30, 2020

No one said college was easy, especially living in a pandemic where hugs are a weapon and a mask is the difference between life and death. I hate it. I hate that there was a possibility of this never occurring.

Week 1 down. Online College: 1 Franny: 0. Content: doable; Motivation: non-existent. As a result of the first week of e-campus, many variables have been brought to the table. Online school is not a good fit for an angsty individual who solely depends on a structure fit for visual learners. Tune in next week for a firsthand look at the pitfalls of online schooling vs. an anomaly, with high hopes that others feel the same.

Frances R.
October 1, 2020

2020 is a dumpster fire. No amount of water can put it out.

Anya R.
October 1, 2020

In the classes I have attended remotely, students seem apprehensive about responding to questions and commenting on class topics. There is a large difference socially between taking a class in person versus taking it remotely. I myself even feel a little weird speaking in class and having my camera on. With the COVID rates rising again, I am nervous that I may not get to attend any of my classes in person.

Brendon R.
October 1, 2020

try and choose to look at this pandemic as an opportunity. Quarantine was definitely a big challenge for me. I am a social person and it was difficult barely having any social interactions. Instead of doing nothing with my time at home I decided to challenge myself by working on my own inner struggles. My main goal was to find comfort in the discomfort. To do this, I would put my phone away during the day so I could stay more in the present moment; rather than distracting myself by looking at other people's lives, I spent time by myself: hiking, swimming in the river, paddle boarding, painting, reading, and journaling. Reflecting back on my goal to find comfort in the discomfort I feel like I made an enormous amount of progress. I am proud of myself for using that time to grow.

Mckenzie M.
October 1, 2020

" So we're following arrows and the flight of the crow"
People tend to follow the lead of those that come before us. Our problem now is that no one has come before us. So we follow what lead we can figure out, leaving us scattered and unsure of what we really "should" be doing. It is easier to leave the questions in the dust and make our own answers for what is safe, easier to follow the people in front of us, regardless of whether their ideas are backed by evidence.

"Living wide screen but what good is it though"

It's easy to say that it's better to look at life's trials objectively, but it often has the side effect of disregarding emotions. We are more than our situation—looking at life objectively just doesn't work all of the time. I could dissect the past week to a point where it has everything to do with the pandemic, but I'd rather focus on the school side of things that has taken over the majority of my thoughts and time.

"When life gets narrower the further you go"

Life continues to present us with challenges, no matter how far we get along in life. There is never a point where you've fully "made it." Sure, milestones can be wonderful, but there is always another challenge just around the corner—another layer to the lives we live.

"Suns set before they rise"

But there will always be more light; our challenges define us no more than our situations do.

Lyrics from "Flight of the Crow" *by Passenger*

Alexis D.
October 1, 2020

It's odd realizing that I have only been seeing half of people's faces on campus because they are wearing masks, and it makes me think about what the rest of their face looks like.

Karina H.
October 2, 2020

There really is no college in COVID-19. It may still exist in some reduced form, but it isn't truly a college. Something is wrong. You can just feel it in class, when you go to get your food, when you try to fall asleep at night. It feels like a hastily cobbled facsimile. It has an artificiality that pervades every sense of this school, interfering with academics and friendships. We keep each other at an arm's length, not able to see each other's faces, a literal mask hiding our humanity. Perpetually hidden in the back of our minds is a caution: "Could this person be the one?" The one who brings this whole experience tumbling down around my ears? We wonder if it's even worth trying to put the effort in to make friendships; we won't ever be able to see each other anyway. Besides, we could get shut down next week. College is not just academia; it is a community. A community of diverse and ambitious people who come together at this place in space and time to step into their future. This year, we lack that community, that connection and solidarity with one another.

Spencer V.
October 4, 2020

COVID-19 Poem

I miss you Abuelo.

It sucks you left us this way.

At the hands of this virus.

Even though I never got to meet you physically, I always miss the calls we had over FaceTime.

You were a great inspiration to me. A true one-of-a-kind human being.

Even though you're gone, you'll always be here.

Where it matters the most.

In my heart.

Rest in Peace Grandpa

Descansa en Paz Abuelo

Gulian C.
October 4, 2020

Sometimes it's hard to love one another when there's not a lot of love going around. In my opinion it's not that hard to put on a mask when it is so simple yet it can save so many lives.

It has become such a political statement, and it is really sad.

Elliana B.
October 4, 2020

As I write this, I sit at my desk, which has become an extension of myself and one of the largest parts of my life due to COVID. This beautiful cherrywood workspace is where I spend most of my time, both as a student and as a young adult. It's where I connect with teachers and friends or spend time alone. This desk is where I go to relax, but also where I go to work. It's become the center of my world, even as my mind dreams of greener pastures. Everything I need is either right here or a few steps away. I have water, paper, knick-knacks, books, my computer, lights, medical supplies, decoration, a plant, important documents, and even board games. The only things I *need* to leave my desk for includes food, water (which can be stored at my desk via water bottle), and the restroom.

But despite the convenience and utility of my desk, I've come to dread it. I don't even want to sit down to message a friend or play a video game anymore because of how much I hate spending my time here. I've been finding myself prioritizing anything and everything other than computer work. I feel like I've memorized every bump and mark on the wall behind my computer. Even though my desk remains as messy as ever, I know where everything is— from the bottle cap just behind my computer monitor to the bank statement in the middle of a stack of papers. I loathe the desk chair I sit in, I dislike the sound of my computer fan, and I've even found myself insulting my desk plant. The monotony is making me go insane. But what else am I supposed to do?

Nathan S.
October 4, 2020

spent a lot of my day on the phone today. My younger brother wanted to tell me all about how he went to the pumpkin patch with my mom and had a blast. My older sister and I chatted about one of our favorite books, *Inkheart*. She went and bought a new copy, as the one we already have is falling apart at the seams. I talked with a few friends from my high school and was reminded of how much I miss them. By noon, my social battery was drained before I even considered exiting my dorm room. It's been strange over the summer and into the fall, not being able to go see friends in-person. I don't want to get used to only video calls.

Hope S.
October 4, 2020

These last couple weeks have been almost dream-like. Everyday feels like a carbon copy of the last. Wake up, shower, eat, go to my room, attend class, spend hours on my phone, eat dinner, and to top it off more phone time until I can't keep my eyes open anymore. Rinse and repeat. It's been the same routine since quarantine started. I was so excited at first; five months of summer, five months of freedom. That anticipated freedom turned into total monotony. Needless to say, I'm ready for change, something I've always been afraid of I want now more than ever. I thank these months of repetition for that. I feel ambitious and ready for something new, something I haven't felt in a long while.

Trey P.
October 5, 2020

My friend in London got COVID at college and had to go home. She told me her other roommates got it too. It's scary to know she got sent home and how there is a possibility it will spread to her family. It also scares me knowing that it can happen to any of us. This week, I've been seeing a lot of people out and about without social distancing. I feel a little worried seeing this because I do not want things to get worse. This week, my other friend in college who is part of a sorority got COVID also. My friend and everyone in the house are all in quarantine. Looking around at other colleges and schools that are being shut down doesn't surprise me, but it also makes me wonder if that will end up happening to us.

Mckenzie M.
October 5, 2020

ately, leaving my house to go to the grocery store is the highlight of my day. (Is that sad or what?) I seriously plan my whole day around it because I get so excited just to leave my house.

Maya B.
October 6, 2020

The smoke rolled in again today. I looked outside this morning and got so excited because I thought it was rain clouds. The smoke is just heavy enough to bother my throat and lungs. So now I feel a little sick but I know it's completely due to the little bit of smoke that's hanging out. However, everyone else doesn't know that so I have to stifle coughs whenever I'm out so no one thinks I've got the Rona.

Alexandria M.
October 8, 2020

What will the end of the pandemic look like? This question has been in my head for quite some time. Will it be soon? Will there be a nationwide announcement, or will it never really go away like the common cold or the flu? I wonder what will happen when everything opens up and there will be a less intense emphasis on delivery systems. Will there be a historic moment where the majority of Americans will leave the country on vacation? It's impossible to foresee what will happen, but it's hard to imagine the switch.

Wyatt D.
October 8, 2020

long for the day when the pandemic is over: when we can spend time with our families and other loved ones (especially our immunocompromised ones); someday we can go on vacation again; when we can go home for Thanksgiving without worrying that we're going to spread the virus and potentially harm someone; when people aren't dying anymore.

Elliana B.
October 11, 2020

In all honesty, perhaps the first thing I notice about college in COVID is how little activity there is. I get up, shower, shave, brush my teeth, and sit in front of a computer the rest of the day. Have you ever tried making connections through a computer screen? Try it sometime. You probably won't be able to—I wasn't. Very quiet, the dorms are mostly silent, at most you see one other person, probably walking away from you. Dinner is the only time there's some human connection. I like dinner.

Spencer V.
October 11, 2020

Recovery

This week I had all four impacted wisdom teeth removed, and for the first time since the pandemic started, I questioned if I would survive if I got COVID-19. Before this surgery I believed myself healthy enough to overcome the flu-like disease. But as I was lying in bed, I didn't feel strong at all. Sure, beforehand I was still wearing masks and trying to avoid spreading the virus, because I believed it was logical to do so. But after getting a sniffle during my recovery, I realized how terrified I was of getting a potentially life threatening cold while my immune system was compromised. It changed my perspective.

Nathan S.
October 11, 2020

This week I have learned a few things:

1. I now completely understand why so many people drop out of college.
2. Insulin is as cheap as water. (I'm being sarcastic.)
3. My boyfriend gives the best hugs.
4. I can't wait to become a teacher and help mold little brains.
5. Weighted blankets and lots of ice cream will get me through college.

Anya R.
October 11, 2020

'm really enjoying the cooler weather. Fall is definitely my favorite season, temperature-wise. Yesterday I ate a bagel with cream cheese and really enjoyed it so I made a second one, which was even better, so I had to make a third. I felt kinda sick after that and took a really long nap. When I woke up, I brushed my teeth and then went to bed. Bit of a nighttime nap if you will. Today I went to Jamba Juice which was really great because I haven't been there in what feels like a few years. I had to get that Purple Dinosaur off the secret menu; so good. I'm feeling pretty decent overall—a little bored but not terrible—just getting by. I hope things change soon, and I'm not necessarily referring to COVID, I just want change. Peace.

Trey P.
October 11, 2020

I wish I could live forever, if only to learn about everything that's ever happened or will happen. I know it's cliché, and I understand the trope that those who attain transcendency find existence meaningless, but I already find existence to be mostly meaningless. The knowledge that someday I will die, well before I have any significant understanding of the world, is a scary thought that invades my consciousness daily. The knowledge (or more accurately, the belief) that all human knowledge will be lost once we cannot adapt to our environment any more is another huge downer. Everything we have done to progress in any way is simply for the sake of progression. None of it will ever last, everything we've done will collapse and be forgotten. The only meaning, therefore, is finding meaning in relationships and knowledge. Making sure that everybody feels loved and comfortable should be the ultimate goal of humanity, even if it will never last. Obtaining the knowledge, and therefore the ability, to do so is equally important, even if all our knowledge is lost when the virtual Library at Alexandria inevitably burns. Unfortunately, people have an innate desire to only care for themselves (and by extension, those they love; a.k.a. those who provide them significant reinforcement). Therefore, we feel a need to hoard knowledge and other resources, alienating everyone outside our circles of reinforcement in the process. This is the pillar of politics. Some find reinforcement from helping others like themselves, others find reinforcement helping those less fortunate. But in the end, we all seek endlessly after our own reinforcement and validation.

Jordan L.
October 11, 2020

Fall is finally almost here and Summer is on its way out. I am noticing the change in colors and the weather is starting to get colder too finally!

Salvador L.
October 11, 2020

attended my grandfather's funeral this week. He died of the virus. No comment.

Susan G.
October 11, 2020

One of the many things that I turned to when quarantine first started back in April was nature. I've lived here in Bend my whole life, and I never experienced the beauty of Central Oregon. For the first time, I went to Shevlin Park, where I truly felt like I was in the outdoors. I could feel the breeze of the Deschutes River blowing across my face, and the air smelled like pine trees. During my hike, I also saw many animals for the first time up close. I saw two rattlesnakes and dozens of birds I've never seen. I know it sounds corny, but to me it was an exciting new experience in nature. The experience led me to buy a kayak to float the river with. It's funny how indoor people (like me) were locked inside, and we turned to nature for activities and recreation for enjoyment. I believe it changed me for the better because I spend lots of time outside now either hiking, biking, or floating the river instead of being inside, playing video games, and watching TV.

Gulian C.
October 13, 2020

Thinking about all the changes that have taken place since COVID and the lockdown started has made me wonder what life will look like when society goes back to normal. Technology has taken over and is essential for our day to day lives now. For example, school is online for the most part. I wonder if we will still use Zoom when COVID is over? Maybe if students are sick and cannot come into school, we won't have to miss a day and can just come to class on Zoom. I also wonder if people will wear masks in public still or if we will take health precautions more seriously. Personally, I believe people will be more sanitary, for example: wash their hands more often, sanitize and clean more. What I have learned from COVID is that there are tiny things we can do to prevent ourselves from getting sick and moving forward I will be more mindful and aware of what I can do to keep myself healthy.

Mckenzie M.
October 13, 2020

Masks

The filter between sane and sick
A metaphor for public safety
A reminder to brush your teeth
An omen of the world today
Masks keep us safe from others
They are the face of the public
Masks are a step towards curing your country
They are a statement
Masks are not a choice
They are mandatory
Masks are a societal duty
They keep us safe
Masks are here to stay
Are you wearing your mask?

Wyatt D.
October 17, 2020

"We can lose and call it living"

Life wouldn't be life without ups and down, without plusses and minuses. Life wouldn't be life without struggle intertangled with happiness. The parts of life that try to pull me down are the moments that make life what it is, make the small moments worth celebrating.

Lyrics from "Call It Dreaming" *by Iron & Wine*

Alexis D.
October 17, 2020

Today I was talking to a friend about our dorms and how it would have been sharing a room with someone else. This led me to wonder who my roommate would have been. After the conversation I began to reminisce about what I imagined college to be like. I never expected it to be like this. Who knew we would not have a roommate, or be sitting in our dorms for class? I feel sad sometimes when thinking about how I thought college would be, however with time I have begun to accept that this is the new reality. In some ways it is nice to have a room to myself and have more than enough space. Although it does get lonely sometimes, and it would be nice to have more company. I am curious to know if next year will be any different. Will we have a roommate? Will COVID still have an impact on our world? Will classes still be on Zoom? I still feel uneasy not knowing the answer to these questions. Despite my worries, I know I can only do what is in my control and I plan on continuing to adapt to my new sort of lifestyle.

Mckenzie M.
October 20, 2020

went swimming this morning and after I got out, I went to walk into the building and had to stop really hard at the door and dig through the pocket of my bag to grab my mask and I got the string caught on the pop socket on my phone and almost flung it on the concrete. But thank goodness I managed to get it on my wet face and #SaveLives.

Alexandria M.
October 21, 2020

VOTED!!! This was my first year being able to vote and I was so excited to be able to do my own research and figure out my own opinion on big kid stuff. I was let down though when I found out I do not get a sticker for voting because honestly that's what I was most looking forward to. I believe they didn't do the voting booth to avoid that human contact for COVID but I was still disappointed.

Ashton K.
October 28, 2020

This week everyone living in the residential hall received an email informing us that a wastewater sampling indicated that COVID-19 could possibly be present in the residence hall. When I saw this email, I was a little worried to know that COVID was in the presence of our campus. At the time I got the email, I was two hours away and I was told the school needed my immediate participation in testing. The email stated that if I was not able to attend by 8 p.m. I would have to go into fourteen days of quarantine. This definitely sparked my anxiety because I do not think I could handle being alone for so long. Luckily, I was given the option to come in the next day and get tested before the other students' tests were sent out. When I went to get tested, it reminded me of how real COVID is. The test this time was different from the one I took when I first arrived at OSU. Instead of having to completely put it up my nose I now did not have to put it up as far. I was glad to hear I did not have to worry about as much discomfort. After my test, I was told I would receive my results in roughly two days. For the past day, I have been more on edge and more mindful of the things I am touching and washing my hands more frequently throughout the day. I am hopeful my results will come back negative because neither myself nor anyone I have been in contact with has experienced symptoms.

Mckenzie M.
October 29, 2020

Right now, it's pretty late and I've been in my dorm room all day working on some homework. I decided not to go out tonight. I really don't have anywhere I would go anyways. My friends came to visit me earlier this week. We had a lot of fun. I would hang out with my friends in the evening after I finished all of my work and we'd just drive around and find things to do. It was fun to see them and be around people from home again. Now it's back to doing homework. I haven't painted in a while and I really want to, I'm just hoping all of my midterms go well.

Allison B.
October 31, 2020

After checking social media yesterday, I'm shocked that my generation (or to be specific, people my age) aren't smart enough to NOT attend parties because of COVID. Like, guys, it's only one day out of the year! Let's be patient and socially distance until this is over! I just can't wrap my head around their logic. Most of us have middle-aged parents, some with parents who have underlying health conditions! Is one day really a fair trade with possibly getting sick? Come on guys.

Gulian C.
November 1, 2020

My first term of college is progressing along, but I don't feel like I'm moving with it. It's almost like the school year is just happening to me. I can't quite tell what I'm struggling with that's based on COVID and what is just college. Am I really bad at being a student or being a virtual student?

Lucy F.
November 1, 2020

This last weekend I went to Eugene to visit my best childhood friend. Lane County currently has the most COVID cases in the state and it was very overwhelming to be in the same environment. I ended up going to Corvallis for the night instead with my best friend and her roommates and felt a bit better about being out and about. While it was fun while the weekend lasted, the anxiety that came after was not pleasant at all. Recently it has been hard to find a balance in my life between being cautious and living my life. A big part of me wants to continue to be safe and distance myself for the sake of my family's health and my personal health, at the same time I am a normal young adult who misses human interaction and going out to socialize in large groups. Socializing is a part of life and key to creating connections in success. Social interactions help one navigate the world and how it operates and eliminates loneliness, an embedded human fear. I hope things ease and it is easier to make a decision that isn't threatening to anyone's health.

Frances R.
November 1, 2020

With everything terrible going on, sometimes it's nice to focus on the positive. We get to spend quality time with a set amount of people. Allowing us to get closer. Some people learn better in a remote setting. I personally love it. We get to focus more on the things we want to, like baking. But then reality sets in. Two hundred thousand people. More people than can sit in a football stadium.

Elliana B.
November 1, 2020

We survived another week! I have to admit that this week when we got the email that we all needed to be tested because they found COVID in the wastewater, I was definitely a little nervous. However, I did take two tests this week and they both came back negative, so that's a positive (haha). But on Friday I went to Corvallis to visit one of my friends at the main campus, and I'm definitely a little nervous that I may have gotten the virus from just being in town. I saw a lot of reckless kids (me being one of them at times, to be honest), and the general attitude was just not worrying about it. I'm happy we have testing available on campus and plan to go on Monday morning to get tested. As always, I am keeping my fingers crossed, and maybe next week I'll have a very interesting COVID journal for you.

Nicholas S.
November 1, 2020

Half of living during a pandemic is groaning at other people's stupidity, then wondering how long it will take their stupidity to kill you. I have a friend going to school in Boston. She has taken a COVID test fourteen times since the start of school, isn't allowed to leave campus, and isn't allowed to be in common areas with more than four people. They serve the food to go, and you are supposed to take it back to your dorm room and eat there. I guess life really is a matter of comparison.

Spencer V.
November 1, 2020

This weekend was upsetting for me. One of my friends who lives in the dorms decided to party in Corvallis on Halloween. Not only did he go to two fraternities, he also went to two sororities and an apartment. He also got frustrated with me for not wanting to see him when he got back. I told him that I do not want to be near him until he gets TRACE-tested. This situation and ones like it are really stressful for me. I know that he is not the only one who was irresponsible this weekend, so I am worried about an outbreak. If these kids keep exposing themselves at big campuses and get some of us sick here, I worry that our campus will close. I am starting to have a lot of fun here and will be extremely disappointed if it is cut short because a few of my classmates have no self-control.

William W.
November 1, 2020

Today I was at work when I found out Biden won. We have an iPad in the middle that the orders come up on so we can start making them. For the last few days, we've kept the news in the bottom corner playing in case something happens. I was pouring someone-s drink when I looked in the bottom corner and Joe Biden's face was on it with "President-Elect" as the headline. I started crying, and we all were screaming. I think overall I feel like I can breathe. I'm so happy, but I'm also even happier for people that this election will really have an effect on.

Lauren H.
November 7, 2020

This week I watched as the election unfolded and for the first time saw how our government works and was able to see my vote count.

Ashton K.

November 7, 2020

feel like we are in an endless cycle of isolation. It has been approximately 225 days since COVID came to Oregon. Two hundred and twenty-five days. Some people have completely reinvented themselves in that time. For others, mental health is at an all-time low and it's hard enough to just get out of bed. People have lost loved ones. Friends. Yet, what is it all for? COVID cases are at an all-time high. Nine hundred and seventy-nine new cases in Oregon yesterday. Nine hundred and seventy-nine cases. When we had the stay-at-home order there were less than 100. Something needs to change.

Elliana B.
November 8, 2020

We are over halfway through my first term in college. Midterms are pretty much over at this point, and now it is a matter of keeping my grades up until finals. I think I have gotten to a point mentally where I'm not expecting to learn or to even do well in my classes. I'm just trying to get through it. I know that I really need to fix my thinking before next term, as my classes start to get harder. That seems like a really difficult task, though. I really need to start talking to my therapist more regularly, and I really need to do some "soul-searching." Next term will be just as virtual as this one has been, and I don't think I've gotten any better at virtual learning since this term began. I just don't know how to get better. Keeping on tops of things is becoming increasingly hard, especially when I struggle to even get into some of my classes. I feel like we've been experiencing more and more tech issues and it's starting to wear me down. I'm really not sure where to go from here.

Lucy F.
November 8, 2020

I am beyond ecstatic today . . . WE WON THE ELECTION. My previous anxiety and fears have

been wiped, and I have been feeling a little more hopeful today. I feel as if I can breathe and

that everything might just actually be okay. On another note, I have been implementing the

social dilemma suggestions in my life and have turned off all notifications on my phone besides

iMessage and phone calls. I have set a time limit on my apps, which has helped reduce 40 percent of

my screen time. I'm hoping I see some long-term results in reducing my stress and anxiety that

comes with social media self-evaluation. I'm hoping these results make me less reliant on social

media and more confident in myself and my talents that I haven't utilized yet due to a reliance

on social media. I'm hoping this helps me grow into a much more independent, self-loving,

self-reliant, inspirational woman.

Frances R.
November 8, 2020

I t finally snowed today! As much as I love rainy weather, snow will always be my favorite. My younger sister called me today to let me know that she had gone to Starbucks at least four times today, just to get the holiday cups. She views November 1 as the first day of the Christmas session. I'm kinda glad that I don't have to be at home to see every Christmas decoration go up this week, as I am not one for the big holiday excitement.

Hope S.
November 8, 2020

When we finally beat COVID (assuming this isn't like the Black Plague and decides to stick around for the next couple of centuries), can we call it a win? How many people died? How many are sick? How many recovered that won't ever be the same? I think this is by definition a Pyrrhic victory. Plutarch wrote after the Pyrrhic War, "If we are victorious in one more battle against the Romans, we shall be utterly ruined." (I think; I'm not sure I quoted it correctly.) We haven't won a battle against COVID yet, and we're close to ruined. What the hell does victory bring?

Spencer V.
November 8, 2020

just read about the new Oregon order to shutdown restaurants again starting Wednesday. I think it's a good thing but I honestly don't think it's going to do what it needs to until the whole country takes a pause for a few weeks. I hope it will help though.

Lauren H.
November 13, 2020

This week there has been a lot of change. Kate Brown announced Friday that there will be a "freeze" starting next Wednesday until December 2. I was honestly surprised to hear this, but also relieved that we are taking extra precautions to try and limit the spread of the virus. Some of the changes that are being made are bars and restaurants will be takeout only, all gyms will be closed, no gatherings with more than six people, and grocery stores and pharmacies will have a limited capacity. It slightly worries me that we are slowly enforcing these precautions again, however it is comforting to know we are being extremely cautious. I wish there was something I could do in my control to help businesses and employees that are being impacted. My grandma owns a restaurant and she has shared with me her anxiety about her business and having to be closed. It is without a doubt an extremely stressful time for everyone and I hope we will be able to find solutions to save our economy. I honestly wonder if this "freeze" will only last for two weeks or if it will last longer. My hope is that these changes will prevent the rise in cases and we will be able to completely reopen again when it is safe.

Mckenzie M.
November 14, 2020

A few days ago, I received an email from OSU that talked about Kate Brown's announcement and going home for Thanksgiving. It said that if students plan on going home for the holidays we should stay at home and not return until the winter term starts. This gave me a lot to think about. I am debating on whether to stay at school for Thanksgiving or go home. I completely understand this decision and think it is smart. I know my family wants me to come spend Thanksgiving with them, and I want to just as much as they do. However, I also do not want to stay at home for a month, I would much rather be at school. I have started to become more worried about the second wave of COVID-19, especially after hearing about businesses beginning to shut down. I hope that we will not have to worry about going into quarantine again and that cases will go down with these new precautions. There is so much change happening in our world right now and I think it is important to remember what we are grateful for. I am grateful for having good health and for authority figures who take initiative in making decisions that will keep us healthy.

Mckenzie M.
November 14, 2020

have had a long week of cold-like symptoms and sad feelings regarding what my life might look like in January. Currently, I live in an apartment with one of my best friends in town, attempting online school while managing the many different relationships my life has to offer: grandparents, friends, boyfriend, and my immediate family. As we enter a statewide freeze, I am starting to become stressed and unsure of what life might look like in a month or so. I am scared for the life and well-being of my family and relatives, while I am sad to see my friends and boyfriend possibly leave me in January depending on the state of our country in regard to this pandemic. With life being so unsure, I turn to meditation and the joy in the little things like being able to take a hot shower and make myself tea when I am stressed. Although we are all facing this pandemic, I still feel like the luckiest girl to have a roof over my head, breathe clean air, eat a meal daily and surround myself with the people I love. It is all going to be okay.

Frances R.
November 15, 2020

The coronavirus has caused so many economical, personal, physical and mental problems. I wouldn't wish on my worst enemy to go through this. You just never really know when things are gonna start looking up.

Kennedy M.
November 15, 2020

Today is weird. The future is uncertain with the new rules about the lockdown that starts in a few days. I will now be doing my finals at home because I am going home for Thanksgiving, and they do not want us to come back until the winter term if that is the case.

Annabelle V.
November 15, 2020

Frustration is the only word that comes to mind at this point in the pandemic. It is obvious that it won't go away unless people follow the guidelines set by the government. A mask is not going to kill anybody. COVID already has. It's not a very difficult thing to understand. It is also literally the easiest option to prevent the spread of the virus. People are just so selfish.

Elliana B.
November 15, 2020

t's scary to watch the people get ready to spend holidays with family when the numbers are at an all-time high in the United States. The hard part is that it's understandable. The people at highest risk are the same people who might need the holiday celebrations the most. We've already given up a lot when it comes to limited contact with our families and friends, and it's natural to want to reach out around the holidays.

Alexis D.
November 21, 2020

To Change the Division Bell

Ideas
Now crafted
alone

Discussion
Held
separately

Listening
Reduced to
hearing

Conversations
Now made in a
Post
We mustn't forget
Communication
Solves
Problems,
Talking
Allows for
listening

Expression
Grants
empathy
For change
We must work together,
To reform the division bell

Wyatt D.
November 21, 2020

This pandemic really made me enjoy the little details: the smell of cookies when they are baking in the oven; the cat stretched out baking in the sun; the warmth of the fire in the woodstove; the sound of the rain on the roof. I am a homebody but this virus has led to a whole new level of comfort, and it is amazing. Sometimes we just have to focus on the positive things and not let our worries take over our lives. We need to pay attention to what's happening around us.

Elliana B.
November 22, 2020

'm really excited for this Saturday because I finally get to go home. I miss everybody a lot and I am so excited to see everyone. "m glad that they are giving out free COVID tests this week because I wanted to get one before I go home. Everything here is now completely online and I can't even eat dinner with my friends. I am very ready to get home and see my family rather than being alone in my room all of the time.

Alison B.
November 22, 2020

think it should be required for people in drive-thrus to wear a mask. I think it's weird that I see so many people come through the drive-thru and no one wears one. I think that just shows that there are so many things people know are morally right to do but they won't do it unless they have to because it's a small inconvenience.

Lauren H.
November 22, 2020

This week I spent most of my time in my room, leaving to get food and maybe driving somewhere for coffee but that's about it. I felt so tired all week and for no reason. I got good sleep and wasn't partaking in any rigorous physical activity. But it's not for no reason; I like to tell myself that I feel tired for no reason but I know why I do. Lounging around my room all day spending all that time glued to a screen isn't going to get me energized, and it's not going to build up energy within me—it's just wasting it slowly. I'm going to try to go outside more next week.

Trey P.
November 22, 2020

Have you ever read the *Epic of Gilgamesh*? It's one of the oldest texts we've found, and it is widely regarded as the first work of literature to exist. Put quite simply, it is the story of becoming human, growing from the base and purely natural, to something more. But there's one line that's stuck with me ever since I read it: "Hold my hand in yours, and we will fear not what hands like ours can do." In context, that's the characters readying themselves for destruction. But to me, it speaks about finding community, working together, building, creating, doing whatever hands like ours are meant to do. In these times, that connection seems even more necessary.

Spencer V.
November 22, 2020

This has been a weird week for COVID. Because it is Thanksgiving, everything is a little bit more confusing. I got TRACE-tested a few days ago in preparation but have still not gotten my results back. This is a little bit scary because I have already gotten home and am seeing my family. I am almost positive I will test negative, but it is still stressful not knowing for sure. My stepmom also went to Mexico recently, which seems really irresponsible. She is apparently trying to get tested but cannot make an appointment. This week seems sketchy altogether, but I will get tested when I get back to campus so hopefully everything turns out okay.

William W.
November 22, 2020

Today is Thanksgiving. It is the first holiday this year where families will be traveling to see each other and gathering in large groups. I have no doubt that we are going to see COVID-19 spikes in the coming weeks. It can be really frustrating to me. My job is at risk if the two-week freeze is extended, and I really need the money. I don't want to sound whiny, but it does feel unfair that I could be laid off because other people are being careless. I've been social distancing; I've been wearing my mask. I didn't attend any Halloween parties, or any parties at all. It's frustrating. The people who complain the most about the lockdowns are the ones who are refusing to follow guidelines. It's annoying. If they had been wearing their masks and had taken a tiny break from partying, we would be in much better shape. We could have stopped being locked down months back, but we're still here. I cannot lose my job right now. It's very likely, though, and I don't know if I can receive any unemployment. I should probably look into it, but I'm trying to be optimistic. It's really hard to be optimistic right now.

Lucy F.
November 26, 2020

decided to write this journal entry on Thanksgiving Day to talk about what I am grateful for, as it has been difficult to find things this year that I am positive about. The one thing I have repeatedly found myself grateful for is the chance to spend another year close to home. Back in June, I was convinced I was attending the University of Denver come the fall of 2020. While that was shortly flawed, I was frustrated and confused about what choosing to stay home would have to offer me. At the time, staying in Bend where I have grown up my whole life seemed like a year full of depression and isolation. Now, as months have gone by and it has been a solid year of life turned upside down from this pandemic, I have realized this is exactly where I was meant to be. I have been given another nine solid months in the presence of my family as all of my family live here. Although my parents are divorced and my grandparents are locked away in fear, I have been able to connect with my family in a way I never would have if I had up and left. I have created a true friendship with my fifteen-year-old sister. I have been inspired by the motherly teachings of my mom, and we have grown to be a lot alike. I have saved the relationship with my dad that has hung on by a thread after the spring of 2020, and I have grown to appreciate my stepparents in a brighter manner that I ever thought possible. I get to laugh over the phone about the ridiculousness of social media and election with my grandpa and connect with my grandma about the intricacies of men and marriage. I am beginning to find myself singing along to my favorite songs that once reminded me of the summer of '16 spending the days at the lake with my best friends. I am finding a new love for Bend's beauty as I take myself down long hikes of uncharted territory. I am me again but better. I am grateful for this pandemic in many ways as it has saved my relationships with my family and friends and has taught me to appreciate myself and the little moments that make up life.

Frances R.
November 26, 2020

There seems to be a lot more sickness going around. If it's COVID or not is questionable, but people are less scared of it this time around since we have shut down our whole lives for so many months for this to just get worse again. I am exhausted. I don't want to wear masks. I want to hang out with my friends. I want to go to school. I want to hug my grandma. I want to go to church. I want to go to a restaurant. This needs to be over.

Ashton K.
November 28, 2020

moved out of Bend a week ago, and I thought college students were stupid. Turns out adults are just as stupid—arguably more so! I've actually seen masks made out of lace. "It makes it easier to breathe," she said. Does she not realize that, in the interest of convenience, she has endangered herself and all of us? Is that not a thought that crosses through other people's heads? Do people have any shred of respect left in them?

Jesus. I'm seriously considering becoming a hermit in the Alaskan wilderness somewhere.

Spencer V.
November 29, 2020

After spending Thanksgiving alone in order to be safer and not harm my family, I headed back to the east coast to spend winter break with my mother. The first day I got here, I found out her boyfriend of five years just tested positive for the coronavirus, leaving my mother most definitely with the coronavirus and unfortunately due to my already close contact with her only three hours into getting home, leaving me with the coronavirus. I canceled work and all friends plans for the next two weeks and am experiencing mild symptoms. It's not the worst place to quarantine but a super bummer that I have it. I had spent so much time being so safe and within hours of winter break I had it.

Kiley P.
November 29, 2020

Thanksgiving. (Hurray!) We had dinner with my grandparents and it was really nice. We went over to our cabin in Eastern Oregon and didn't have to deal with COVID mandates of any kind for almost a whole week and it was glorious.

Alexandria M.
November 29, 2020

am so ready for Christmas.

Salvador L.
November 29, 2020

This week has been one of the strangest weeks yet. My dad drove over last Tuesday and picked me up to take me home for Thanksgiving break. Going home was such a strange feeling. I felt like I should be going to parties and seeing all of my old high school friends. But nothing like this was happening this year because of COVID. I only got to see a few of my closest friends that were also home on break. I was planning to play a lot of video games but only hopped on a few times. I have come to value real life interactions over talking with my friends online, especially now when I feel like I never have enough social interactions. The first few days I spent most of my time with my family, because it was good to catch up and hear what they have been up to. After about three or four days I started getting so sick of being home. I remember why I hated it so much; there was never anything fun to do and living at home is not fun. I have become even more grateful for how well Cascades has worked out for me.

Colin B.
November 30, 2020

To wrap my last COVID journal of this term, I just want to give myself a pat on the back for finishing my first term in college during a pandemic. It was definitely a roller coaster when it comes to everything: technology, emotions, and setting meaningful, good study habits. This is a big deal to me, as I'm a first-generation student coming from Mexican immigrant parents who never got to hold a graduation diploma. Just got to keep my head up and look forward to another three semesters this year. Good job, Gulian.

Gulian C.
December 3, 2020

am so tired. Of online school. Of being home. Of the world imploding. I just want normal back. I want to stop the feeling of impending doom.

Alexandria M.
December 4, 2020

Okay, I'm starting to understand quarantine and the public's reaction to it a little bit better now. I'm reading Twain's *What is Man?*, and in the first chapter he makes the case that humans are machines that require experience and situation to form thoughts and opinions. In other words, reality is less something we observe than it is a product of our experiences and perception. Applying this same frame to today's world, it makes individual responses much simpler to comprehend. Because these individuals haven't had the virus touch them personally, it hasn't invaded their reality. No matter how much media or legislation is thrown at them, they exist with a cerebral knowledge of COVID and act as though it were a figment of their imagination. Is that a pain in the ass or what?

Spencer V.
December 6, 2020

Right after I came back to school, my dad tested positive for COVID. This was pretty scary, but he had only mild symptoms and was the only one who got it. I had to quarantine in my room for four days which kind of sucked because I missed my friends and will only be here for two weeks. I tested negative though!!! My friend also told me that a vaccine is coming super soon so that's cool too. It sounds selfish because people have it so much worse than I do, but I really want to be able to do normal stuff again soon.

William W.
December 6, 2020

started college during a global pandemic. How many people can say that? Sometimes it felt like it was so easy to just climb out of bed, turn the computer on, and bam, I was in class. Other times it felt like there was no escaping the stressful reality I was trapped in, four walls surrounding me, a window that appears almost like a television, capturing people walking down the street and snow falling gracefully to the ground. And few moments of fresh air, not because I didn't want to go outside, but the anxiety of leaving the safety of comfort was too much to handle. In reality, I'm still here. I made it. Looking back over the term, I can see that having something that makes you work hard is so important. Over the summer there was nothing to do all day but watch TV and bake. I soon got bored of that, so I began just going through the motions of daily life. Now, dealing with deadlines and pressure from school to work hard, I find myself happier. Even with all of these challenges that are thrown my way. I can really be proud of myself.

Elliana B.
December 6, 2020

Friday, December 4, 2020, was sadly a record-breaking day for COVID-19 cases. It was reported by Oregon health officials that the highest number of daily cases to date is 2,176. This is so sad to me because I feel like we have so little control over the virus. We can only do so much to prevent it, and it is honestly terrifying to think we do not know what we will have to confront next. After Thanksgiving, I came back to campus and am staying here until Christmas break. I did not think there would be any differences when I came back, however I completely forgot that OSU–Cascades students were given the option to stay at home. It is so odd being at school when there is barely anyone around. I do not like how ghost-like it feels in the dorms or how the hallways feel so empty and quiet. It is sad to me the number of people who I have talked to that are moving off campus this next upcoming term due to COVID-19, although I completely understand their reasons for moving. Even though my first term of college has not been what I expected, I am still beyond grateful that I had the opportunity to live on campus.

Mckenzie M.
December 6, 2020

never in a million years would have thought that this pandemic would take up such a big part of my life from my senior year to my freshman year of college, such big milestones that were covered up with fabric on our faces and no celebrations.

Ashton K.
December 6, 2020

I guess this is my last COVID journal entry for the year. I wanted to make this entry a look into what I learned and took from this term in regard to attempting college with COVID-19. When looking back on my weeks of journal entries and weeks of schooling, I notice a lot of growth and self-realization. I entered this school year with a lot of doubt and stress with beginning a school year that was so unknown. There were many variables to online school that I didn't believe I could handle or accomplish: being on top of assignments, creating relationships, and gaining solid knowledge in my classes. I have learned how to work harder in so many ways that resulted in self-growth and hope. I have become more motivated. I have learned plenty but about things that interest me. I have maintained relationships with the ones that matter. I have received outstanding grades. I have become more confident in my work and who I am. I have learned how to get through difficult times and come out the end more positive and grateful. I am grateful for my family, my close friends, my teachers and most of all myself because if it wasn't for my strength and compassion I wouldn't have achieved what I have today. So, thank you COVID for teaching me to find happiness in the moment and not receive everything I wanted but appreciate everything I have.

Frances R.
December 6, 2020

CPSIA information can be obtained
at www.ICGtesting.com
Printed in the USA
BVHW030935161221
624197BV00006B/270